INTERMITTENT FASTING

A Simple, Proven Approach to the
Intermittent Fasting Lifestyle -
Burn Fat, Build Muscle,
Eat What You Want

solely under their purview. There are no scenarios in which the publisher or the original author of this work can be in any fashion deemed liable for any hardship or damages that may befall them after undertaking information described herein.

Additionally, the information found on the following pages is intended for informational purposes only and should thus be considered, universal. As befitting its nature, the information presented is without assurance regarding its continued validity or interim quality. Trademarks that mentioned are done without written consent and can in no way be considered an endorsement from the trademark holder.

Table of Contents

INTRODUCTION

If you are an avid searcher for methods and techniques that you hopefully think would help you
achieve your desired body figure and health, you
might have already run into several terms associated
with diet and workout like Atkins diet, ketogenic diet,
water therapy, and strength training.

There are actually a lot more terms and each of them
probably had become a top searched figure at least
once. But, there is this one method that is becoming
more and more prominent these days, as it continues
to prove its effectiveness not only to weight loss but
also to the overall health of an individual—the intermittent fasting.

What if I told you that losing weight is not necessarily
a matter of "what you eat," but instead a matter of

"when you eat?" In this book, you'll find out what intermittent fasting is, and why people who relied on several diet methods before are gradually moving into this method.

This book will guide you throughout your journey; from learning everything about intermittent fasting up to applying the method to your lifestyle. You'll discover the benefits of the method not only as a way to lose fat but also as a means to improve certain functions in your health. There is also a step-by-step, comprehensive guide that will provide all the help you need so you could start on your new weight-loss program.

Get ready for the huge changes in your lifestyle and be prepared for the massive results that await you, as you take your very first step in this life-changing journey to a healthy weight loss!

FREE BONUS BOOK

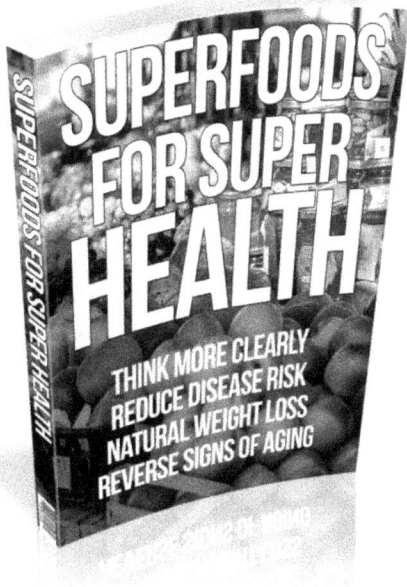

As a Thank You for purchasing this book, I would like to offer you another book as a special bonus! It is called "Super Foods For Super Health".

This comprehensive book is for those who are interested in:

- Learning more about super foods that you can easily get your hands on today.

- How to incorporate those super foods into your everyday meals.

- Nutritional benefits for each super foods

- How to improve your overall health

- How to lose weight naturally

- How to reduce disease risk

- How to reverse signs of aging

- Think more clearly

- Improving your focus

- And much more..

So if you are interested in learning more about any of the above, just go to http://bit.ly/superfoods-gift and grab your free bonus book!

PART I – EVERYTHING YOU NEED TO KNOW ABOUT INTERMITTENT FASTING

CHAPTER 1

THE PRACTICE OF FASTING

Fasting has been one of the most prominent methods of weight loss ever since it was introduced to our history. Up until today, there are a lot of people who prefer using the fasting method to shed some pounds, as they believe it's the best way to lose weight. Some of those who have proven the effectiveness of fasting even call it a "life cheat" or a "life hack" as it provides the result they desire without any cost at all.

There are, however, several claims that discredit the method and prove contrary to what is said to be its effect. Some nutritionists say that fasting is unhealthy and should not be promoted to the public as it can cause nutrition deficiencies and other health-related problems. In spite of this, there are still people who find fasting a great and easy way to lose weight. But, is fasting really just a matter of not eating to reduce body weight?

Fasting, in its purest definition, is the abstinence from consuming foods, drinks, or both for a certain period of time. During the early ages when different religions were still fighting over lands, people, and beliefs, it was not considered a form of diet; but instead, a practice to prove one's faith to the god of whatever religion a man believed. It was more of an obedience rather than a health-related practice.

Nowadays, fasting is still associated with existing religions and is still regarded as a part of religious practices. In Buddhism, monks and nuns strictly abide by the Vinaya rules. They do not eat after the noon meal and they stick to this practice every day. Under Christianity, the practice of fasting is linked to the passages expressly written in the biblical Book of Isaiah. In there, fasting is said to be not only a mere abstinence from food or water but also a decision to fully obey the god's commands. And in Islam, Muslims believe that aside from food abstinence, the practice of "fasting" also entails avoidance of acting and speaking of falsehood.

In the context of physiology and health, fasting refers simply to a person's metabolic status when he has not eaten overnight. It's the metabolic state after a person achieves full digestion and absorption of meal. It usually happens during sleep as this is the phase when the body doesn't receive anything and thus, is focused only on full digestion. From this very description, we can say that fasting is not just one of the thousands of methods of losing weight. It's actually a normal phenomenon that happens to every person, every day.

Just like those of any other practice related to health improvement and diet, the effects of fasting differ from person to person, depending on a variety of factors such as a person's age, current medication he is currently taking, his existing health issues if there are any, and his body's response to hunger. Nonetheless, fasting still has proven its own importance in the field of medicine and medical research.

There are distinguished types into which different ways of fasting are usually categorized namely dry fasting, water fasting, diagnostic fast, and intermittent fasting. All of these types use abstinence from either food or water but vary on their purposes.

Absolute Fast

An absolute fast (also known as dry fasting) is the complete abstinence of food and liquid that lasts commonly for 24 hours. This type of fasting can further be extended up to a couple of days. This is usually a practice done for religious purposes.

Water Fast

This type of fasting is almost like an absolute fasting except that it allows the consumption of drinking water during fasting period; but aside from drinking water, all other liquids are prohibited. This type is believed to be practiced by some people in order to "cleanse" their bodies. The most common diet method associated with this type is the water therapy which has been proven effective in weight-loss procedures.

Diagnostic Fast

Diagnostic fast is a fasting supported by medical practitioners. It is technically a part of medical procedure performed as a pre-observation measure. It is a fasting advised to, and done by people who undergo or will undergo a medical investigation with regard to certain health problems like hypoglycemia. Some procedures also require diagnostic fasting before the actual check-up such as in a colonoscopy.

Intermittent Fast

Intermittent fasting is the type of fasting that is neither absolute nor done for diagnostic purposes. It is seen as an aid in diet and is proven effective for burning fats, building muscle, and controlling nutritional intake. This will be elaborately discussed in the proceeding chapters. There is also a section that will guide you on how to perform intermittent fasting properly and the supplemental things that will help you achieve better results. So, what are you waiting for? Let's proceed to the next chapter!

CHAPTER 2

INTERMITTENT FASTING

They say an apple a day keeps the doctor away, but consuming like seven or more apples each day is not anymore covered by this golden saying.

Eating a lot of healthy foods can surely provide dramatic changes to your overall health. However, "a lot" of these foods could sometimes be "too much" for your body that it wouldn't be able to respond properly anymore; yes, even those foods which are worshipped as the healthiest. This is when intermittent fasting comes in—promoting nutrition regulation and diet control.

But, what exactly is intermittent fasting? Intermittent fasting is an eating or diet schedule which follows a cycle of alternating eating and no-eating periods. A person who practices intermittent fasting basically abides by a schedule that divides the day or the week into fasting and eating periods which are patterned at regular intervals. For example, on a week-based intermittent fasting schedule, a person might assign his Mondays, Wednesdays, and Saturdays as fasting periods, which means he should not eat on those days; and then his Sundays, Tuesdays, Thursdays, and Fridays as his eating periods.

Assigning schedules for intermittent fasting can be as simple as every other day, or as complex as a combination of week-based and day-based fasting—in a day-based fasting, a person splits his daily time frame into eating and fasting periods. In any case, intermittent fasting isn't really that much of a new idea to the body.

As once mentioned in the preceding chapter, the time when a person sleeps can already be considered as fasting time. This is because the body's digestive properties do not have any new substance to digest during sleep; thus, they stop right after fully completing the digestion. The idea of intermittent fasting is simply to extend this portion of time and retain the "empty" state of stomach until the next scheduled eating time. It's almost just like sleeping for a longer period.

How Intermittent Fasting Is Done

Let's say for example, you are planning to start practicing a day-based intermittent fasting. The first thing you want to know is how long your fasting period should be in each day. Ideally, the proper fasting period should be 15 to 16 hours a day; this leaves you nine to eight hours for your eating period. The remaining eight- or nine-hour eating window should strictly be the only time when you are allowed to eat. Majority of those who practice intermittent fasting usually set two meals for this length.

Now that you know both your eating period and fasting period, you need to choose which time should each period start and end. If you are familiar with weight-loss diet plans and protocols, you probably know that the best time at which you can set your dinner is as early as seven or eight in the evening. Let's say that you set your dinner at seven in the evening, counting back eight hours from 7 pm you'll have 11 am. This means that your eating period should start at 11 in the morning and should end at seven in the evening. The rest of the hours that are not covered by your eating window should be a no-eating or -drinking period. If you normally wake up at 8 am then you should skip the breakfast, take your lunch at 11 am, have your dinner at 7 pm and sleep at whatever time you usually go to bed.

Science and Medical Research

Several studies were already done to examine the effectiveness and safety of intermittent fasting. Most of the results of these research studies showed remarks that were close to each other although the proponents and other scientists have not yet come up with a hard and fast conclusion. This is because each result had its own distinct negative impact to the samples; from minor issues to major health problems. Scientists believe that these issues were brought by a lot of factors such as the differences in the health of participants, and the foods, themselves which are offered during eating time. Nevertheless, the positive effects of most of these studies were found to be more dominant than the negative ones. This induces the scientists and researchers to further conduct studies to support this type of fasting.

One of the most prominent and current research done concerning the effects of scheduled or intermittent fasting was a research in endocrinology conducted by proponents from the United States of America. The study called the fasting schedule as intermittent energy restriction or IER. The IER's counterpart was the ad libitum feeding or free feeding. The IER followed the intermittent fasting schedule while the ad libitum feeding simply based the feeding on the sample's own biological hunger phase.

Like in the usual setting of laboratory tests, the first testing was done on rodents. The mice were divided into two groups—the IER group and the free-feeding group. After five months of feeding, both groups were observed and examined. It was found out that among the mice used for testing, those under the IER group showed dramatic reduction from their initial glucose and insulin levels—the examination was a part of a study about type 2 diabetes. Those under the free-feeding group, on the other hand, either retained their original glucose and insulin levels or developed slight changes from their original levels. Either way, it was found out that the glucose and insulin levels of mice in the IER group were significantly lower than those of the mice in the other group.

It was further found out from the same research study that despite having lower glucose and insulin levels, the mice under the IER group were surprisingly not suffering from energy deficiency. The proponents believe that it was because the mice of IER group had already adapted to their new eating setting and they therefore would require only less levels of glucose and insulin intake to suffice their energy needs.

There was also a study that found intermittent fasting as a huge contributory factor when it comes to weight loss. Such study also involved rodents as its subjects. In the first phase of the test, all of the rats had ad libitum access to standard food; they were able to consume meals whenever they felt hungry. The first phase lasted for four weeks. After the fourth week, the rats were then divided into two groups. The first group of rats continued with the ad libitum feeding while the second group underwent strict diet schedule which consisted eating and fasting days, similar to the IER group from the previously mentioned study.

The rats from each group were then further tested for another 10 weeks. After the 10th week, each of the group was examined—it was discovered that there were huge reductions in the body weights of those rats under the second group or the IER group. The differences between the body weights of the rats belonging to the IER group after the first phase of the study and after the second phase, were comparable to those of the rats which belonged to the first group. The results were further examined and brought to an analysis of the IER's efficacy in relation to the development of insulin resistance due to high fat diet.

Intermittent Fasting Effects on Humans

Of course, the previously mentioned pieces of evidence won't be enough to back up even just half of the claimed efficacy of intermittent fasting for these only involved rodents as their subjects. But in the usual research laboratory environment, such tests are relevant and reasonable enough to consider the study as applicable to an upper level form of subject—humans.

One research study featured on an article entitled, Nutrition & Diabetes, suggested that intermittent fasting—coupled with low-energy diet—resulted to improvements on both glucose metabolism and cardiovascular health. The study involved both over-weight and obese people. It used IER trial as well and the observation period lasted three months. After the third month of strict diet implementation, the subjects were examined to identify the presence of cardiovascular risk markers and to assess the glucose levels of individuals.

Majority of the subjects showed positive changes on both aspects. There were less risk markers on their cardiovascular health which could lead to serious heart diseases if left maintained at a high level. Plus, their glucose metabolism has improved. The subjects' levels of blood pressure were also examined in the same study although there were minimal inconsistencies when such results are compared to the results of other studies which also focused on the effects of intermittent fasting. Thus, only the IER's effect on cardiovascular health and glucose properties of humans was considered safe to conclude, at least as of the current state.

There was also an intermittent fasting trial performed on non-obese, healthy individuals. In a matter of three weeks, effects became evident on the in-

dividuals who took part in the trial. On men participants, triglyceride levels were lowered to a healthier
state. Triglyceride is an organic compound which can
be found in a human body. The presence of high levels of triglyceride compounds in the body is a sign
that an individual is prone to or has diabetes or kidney disease.

With regard to the women participants, the researchers found a post-treatment increase in high-density
lipoprotein or HDL cholesterol. HDL cholesterol
functions as an important substance in the body as it
removes excess cholesterol from the blood, the cells,
and the walls of blood vessels; hence, called the good
cholesterol. The variation of the effects based on gender is believed to be caused by the level of fasting
each gender group naturally possesses; men participants tended to have higher fasting levels than
women participants. Though the results of the study
were found to be gender-specific, they were considered a helpful tool to demonstrate the positive effects
of intermittent fasting.

There are more studies to back up the effects of intermittent fasting but enumerating each would take a

lifetime to be thoroughly explained. Besides, the concept of intermittent fasting, being widely accepted as a major topic on health and diet, has just yet begun on getting attention in the field of medical research. That is why the studies related to it are not as numerous and as conclusive as those which have focused on well-known, broader health topics such as diabetes, skin care, or workout trainings.

CHAPTER 3

BENEFITS OF INTERMITTENT
FASTING

Even if intermittent fasting sounds like a common practice that has been naturally existing for centuries, the conceptualization of the practice is actually not that old. A number of research studies are still on the line and medical researchers are still either planning or conducting several trials in pursuit of developing a solid conclusion to close the case—which would be more likely to take years or decades to happen.

But as of the studies that are currently on record, intermittent fasting already holds quite a decent impression when it comes to human health. Majority of the past trials ended up with a positive conclusion regarding the beneficial effects of the diet concept to people. These benefits include induced cell repair processes, reduced oxidative stress, lowered insulin resistance, increased brain function and protection, weight loss and muscle growth, as well as increased protection against certain diseases.

Induced Repair Processes on Cells

Fasting prompts the cells in your body to perform autophagy which is the process through which cells undergo self-destruction. Autophagy is a normal physiological phenomenon which is meant to maintain normal cellular functioning. Destroyed cell organelles are turned over for the generation of new cells. This helps the body maintain a healthy set of cells and get rid of unnecessary or damaged organelles which could cause serious diseases such as cancer, when not destroyed.

When an individual does not consume food or water for a prolonged span of time, the stress level in his body increases. A healthily elevated stress level induces autophagy to take place; and this is the exact reason that fasting is considered a biological stressor which brings a healthy amount of positive effects in the body including autophagy.

Reduced Oxidative Stress

Oxidative stress happens when the production of free radicals is not countered by the body's ability to detoxify their negative effects to health. This happens either because there is an abnormally excessive production of free radicals that the body's natural ability, even at a normal state, cannot battle the free radicals' harmful effects; or because the body's antioxidant activity became too weak that it couldn't keep pace even with the normal production of free radicals.

The ability of the body to deter harmful effects of free radicals is called neutralization which is brought by the body's antioxidants. Antioxidants are molecules that safely interact with free radicals, as well as counteract and detoxify their harmful effects, to maintain a healthy set of cells. An imbalance between antioxidant activity and free radical production brings oxidative stress to place; and therefore, damages the components of the cell.

Short-period fasting works by ironically causing a slight increase in free radical production. This triggers the cells in the body to respond on a more secure level by increasing the level of anti-oxidant activity. When this happens, the antioxidants will be able to detoxify all the free radicals and will lessen the oxidative stress.

Lowered Insulin Resistance

Insulin is a hormone produced by the pancreas which extracts glucose from carbohydrates and converts them into energy. It can also store glucose in the body for future use. However, when the body receives too much insulin, it tries to counter this excessive level until it eventually fails to respond properly to the hormone.

Insulin resistance is a serious complication that entails some of the known major health problems. This is because insulin helps keep the body's blood sugar level in regulation. Thus, when the body resists insulin, it also loses its control over blood sugar level; making the body prone to both hyperglycemia or the surge in blood sugar level, or hypoglycemia or the abnormal drop in blood sugar level.

In a certain study involving humans as subjects, intermittent fasting was attributed to a 3-6% decrease in blood sugar and 20-31% drop in insulin level. The figures showed good indications of insulin level improvement. A decrease in insulin level is technically helpful since in the first place, insulin resistance is brought by excessive insulin level. The study also showed that intermittent fasting protected the subjects from kidney damage.

Increased Brain Function and Protection

As of the currently existing studies, though only involving animal samples, intermittent fasting has proven a number of benefits to the brain. One of these studies discovered that the growth of nerve cells on those mice which underwent intermittent fasting, accelerated after the intervention period. Another study showed that intermittent fasting could prevent brain damage that could further lead to stroke.

An increase in brain-derived neurotrophic factor or BDNF was also found evident on the samples involved in a study about dietary restriction and its effects on the brain. Deficiency in BDNF hormones are implicated in various mental health issues including depression.

Weight Loss and Muscle Growth

Among the effects of intermittent fasting, weight loss is what people sought after the most. This type of diet pattern has been used and incorporated in several fitness plans and is becoming more and more trendy among health-conscious people because of its huge impact to the body. Plus, it comes with a bonus— studies show that intermittent fasting helps retain lean mass and promote muscle growth. All of these will be elaborately discussed in the next chapter.

Increased Protection Against Certain Diseases

Due to the previously mentioned benefits, it is apparent that intermittent fasting can safely be attributed to lowered risks of certain types of diseases. The improved cell repair processing can help the body get rid of cancer. The decrease in oxidative stress may battle brain-health issues such as depression and Alzheimer's disease. Improvements in insulin level, on the other hand, are directly connected to insulin resistance and are therefore helpful to combat diabetes as well. Above all, intermittent fasting is an effective tool for a healthier way of losing weight, making it both a preventive and a corrective measure against obesity.

INTERMITTENT FASTING – KEY TO A HEALTHY WEIGHT LOSS AND MUSCLE GROWTH

The most probable reason a person follows an intermittent fasting schedule is weight loss. Fortunately, weight loss is among one of the evidence-supported benefits that intermittent fasting promotes. Well, fasting in general promotes weight loss; so, what makes intermittent fasting a different and better option?

When you fast, you basically do not allow your body to receive calories from foods. This means you are not prone to storing excess calories as fats in your body. Therefore, if your body continues to fast, there are only two things that can happen to your body weight—remain as is or decrease. Among the two, it is the latter which is more likely to happen since fats are naturally burned during activities regardless if they are eventually replaced or not.

Although the idea is scientifically true, not all people who tried fasting succeeded in losing weight. As a matter of fact, some of them even ended up gaining more. This is because the general term "fasting" simply means abstaining from foods, drinks, or both. It does not define how much to abstain, for how long one should abstain, nor what happens next after someone starved himself for an unusual length of time—it often ends up being misinterpreted as an un-regulated way of skipping at least one full meal.

Most of the people "fast" by skipping breakfast. But when the lunch time comes, they tend to eat more than usual to satisfy the prolonged hunger they endured before the meal. This is the common mistake people do when they fast; they do not pair it with dis-cipline. If you fast for 48 hours, you'll most probably eat a lot on your next meal as your body needs to gain what it didn't during the fasting period; regardless if you try to control it or not. This is why fasting for straight long periods is not recommended by nutritionists and health experts.

Intermittent fasting, on the other hand, follows a uniform cycle of periods; hence, regulated. It gradually lets the body adjust into a new setup until it becomes used to it. It does not abuse hunger too much as it still includes the three main meals of the day, or two at the least. So, there is nothing to worry about not being able to control food intake. The diet concept actually just expands the span of time when your body is not consuming anything and narrows your eating-window. This is considerably a healthy setup if you want to shed some pounds. In here, you are giving your body enough time to fully digest meals so as to absorb the nutrients properly instead of merely storing them as fats.

Accelerated Fat-Burning Process

Moreover, short-period fasting also accelerates your metabolism which means your body can burn more calories when you follow intermittent fasting. In a certain study published by the National Center for Biotechnology Information or NCBI in the US National Library of Medicine, short-term starvation led to an average of 3.6% increase in the metabolic rate of the subjects.

11 healthy young individuals took part in the said study, all of whom are normal-weight. They were not allowed to eat meals for 48 hours. After the intervention period, the metabolic rate of each individual increased in varied rates with a mean of 3.6%. Such number was considered as a large increase in metabolism level and was entirely attributed to the starvation or fasting period.

Intermittent Fasting vs. Daily Calorie Restriction

There exists a traditional diet regimen called daily calorie restriction or CR through which an individual limits his daily calorie intake to a fixed measure. If you adopt this kind of diet technique, you need to be conscious on the quantity of the food you consume and make sure that you do not exceed your calorie limit. So, if let's say, you are only allowed to take 1500 calories per day, your total calorie consumption should not be 1600 or 1700 calories but 1400 calories or below are allowed. This technique has proven favorable results to individuals who practice the CR method but there's one downside to this—it's hard to maintain such kind of diet.

First of all, the meals an individual takes every day usually do not have a readily available calorie measure. And in such case, the individual must rely heavily on estimation which is not a good thing, considering that the very purpose of the CR method is to quantify the exact calorie intake of a person in order to regulate consumption. Unfortunately, approximation is not ideal most especially when you need to implement the diet method in the strictest terms.

Secondly, even if an individual consumes foods and products in boxes or cartons (which most probably have a calorie amount indicator on their nutrition facts sections), it will be hard for an individual to guarantee that what he had just consumed would be equal to the calorie amount that was written on the packaging; say, what if he did not consume all the content? Besides, packed foods are not really the healthiest option for an individual who claims to be "on a diet."

Lastly, it's not always safe to say that a person can control his food intake every day based on a fixed calorie limit. It should not be forgotten that calories are also energy providers and not just "potential" fats. There might come a day which would demand more energy from an individual and choosing to stick with the limited-calorie food intake clearly would not be efficient.

In contrast to the quantified restriction of CR method, intermittent fasting allows free intake of food during eating-windows. This diet schedule is after the lengthening of fasting period and shortening the eating period without necessarily limiting the calorie intake; while the CR method does not restrict consumption based on time but on the size of food, itself. To be honest, both are equally effective in reducing weight but there are recent studies which can back up the claim that intermittent fasting is better than calorie restriction method in some aspects other than mere fat mass reduction.

According to an article published by the Department of Kinesiology and Nutrition of the University of Illinois in Chicago, the intermittent diet schedule may be more effective in retaining the lean mass in the body while reducing weight. The study used obese individuals as subjects. The review focused on examining weight loss as well as the corresponding fat mass loss and lean mass retention. Under the daily CR diet, the average weight loss was 5-8% while the average fat mass loss was 10-20%. On the other hand, the intermittent diet resulted into 4-8% average weight loss and 11-16% fat mass loss.

The figures were evidently near to each type. However, the researchers further identified that although both were effective for weight reduction, the intermittent fasting resulted to a greater retention of lean mass than CR diet. Lean mass, in a nutshell, is the portion in your weight that isn't fat. This portion includes the weight of your bones, your muscles, the water in your body, and technically, all of your organs. This is the reason that a lot of nutritionists advise body builders to go after either retaining or gaining lean mass while reducing fat mass.

Muscle Mass Retention and Growth

An unregulated fasting might be helpful in losing weight but the problem with it is that along the process of shedding fat mass, you might also lose some of your lean mass. This is a crucial matter as a lot of people mistake losing weight as synonymous to being healthy. Unless all the weight you lost is composed of fat mass, it is not safe to say that your body did get healthier.

It is only important to understand that fat loss is different from muscle loss although the tricky part is that, both can happen in a single weight loss activity. If you focus too much on losing weight without keeping track of your muscle health, chances are you'll end up degrading your muscle strength. Since intermittent fasting helps retain lean mass amid weight reduction, it can therefore also help retain muscle mass for body builders.

Retaining muscle mass is just as hard as gaining it. Even if you gained much, it won't make any noticeable change if you also lost much of it at the same time. Let's say for example, you weigh 170 pounds and that you constantly gain two pounds of muscle mass per month because of consistent training. In a span of one year, we can say that you'll gain 24 pounds of lean muscle mass turning your initial 170-pound weight into 194 pounds. That is a huge muscle improvement considering you didn't gain any significant fat mass the whole year. But what if during the year, due to unregulated fasting, you also lost a total of 23 pounds of lean mass? Your weight at the end of the year will then only be 171 pounds—a frustratingly one-pound gain for a whole year of training.

Consistency in growth is the key to build stronger muscles—and to look more ripped in case appearance is a factor. This is why muscle gainers must follow diet patterns which support retention of lean muscle mass. And such rule shall also apply to those who want to lose weight and gain muscle at the same time.

Getting Rid of Belly Fat

If you are one of those people who are overly conscious with their fat tummies and how they keep on showing a bump under your otherwise gorgeous clothes, then there's a good news for you—intermittent fasting is also associated with belly fat reduction.

There was a study regarding the effect of intermittent fasting on type 2 diabetes, which tested individuals with "fat tummies." These individuals underwent intermittent fasting and after 24 weeks, the fasting alone provided the individuals 4-7% waist circumference reduction. This is largely connected to the previously tested efficacy of intermittent fasting when it comes to overall weight loss.

CHAPTER 5

TYPES OF INTERMITTENT FASTING

Several variations of intermittent fasting have already been made even before the diet pattern became popular to the world. And as it gets more and more attention from health enthusiasts and nutritional experts, the list becomes longer. All of the types that exist to date are created out of varying needs so it cannot really be identified which among these "best" fits all. In fact, majority of those who largely benefited from intermittent fasting are using a mixture of two or more of these types.

There are, however, a few types of intermittent fasting that have established a decent impression to both nutritionists and diet experts. These intermittent fasting variants have made it to the list mainly because a number of people found these diet patterns appropriate for them and for their needs.

5:2 Diet

Popularized by British journalist and producer Michael Mosley, this is by far the most prominent kind of intermittent fasting. 5:2 diet is a week-based fasting schedule meaning; a cycle lasts for a week and every cycle or week is split into fasting and eating days. This is a simple schedule that can be followed by anyone and is also among one of the most flexible diet patterns.

5:2 basically means five whole days of free-eating for two full days of fasting. Since a week is composed of seven days, you can just set two of these days as your fasting days and freely consume foods for the rest of the week. On every fasting day, you can only consume a total of not more than 25% of your average daily calorie consumption. Yes, "fasting" here refers to a period of limited intake and not an absolutely no-food nor -drink period; thus, you can still eat but with limitation.

To provide a clearer picture of how 5:2 diet is followed, let's say you designated your Wednesdays and Thursdays as your fasting days. On your Fridays up to your Tuesdays, you can eat your meals the way you normally do; you can eat breakfast, lunch, dinner and even snacks. There are no limits on eating days. On the other hand, your Wednesdays and Thursdays are a little stricter when it comes to your consumption. If your average calorie consumption per day is let's say 2000, your calorie limit would be 500 (2000 multiplied by 25%). This means you should not eat more than 500 calories on your Wednesdays and neither on your Thursdays. Fasting days in 5:2 diet aren't that strict though. You can still have three meals during these days except that the meals would be relatively smaller.

Do your fasting days have to be consecutive days? Well, as stated earlier, 5:2 diet is known for being one of the most flexible diet patterns; so nope, those days do not necessarily have to be consecutive. Majority of the 5:2 diet users find hunger easier to sustain when the two fasting days are apart from each other like Mondays and Wednesdays or Tuesdays and Fridays. It is even highly recommended for beginners to set these periods on non-consecutive days, considering a

75% decrease in one's normal calorie intake is a huge, sudden drop. So, if you want to overcome your first few weeks under 5:2 diet, better refrain from picking two consecutive days. Consecutive days are more convenient though and as long as the fasting won't exceed 48 hours, they are believed to provide equally healthy but slightly faster results.

Another thing that makes it a flexible diet pattern is that each cycle does not have to follow a uniform pattern. This means you can fast on the Thursday and Friday of the current week and switch these fasting days into the Tuesday and Wednesday of the following week. Of course, uniform cycles are better so your body could adapt to consistency but it's much better to stick to reality and consider the possibilities that you can't always be free to fast on the same days of every week. Nonetheless, it is still up to you how you would like to apply this type of intermittent fasting to each of your weeks.

Further, some of the other types of intermittent fasting were actually just variations of the 5:2 diet. There is also a 4:3 diet which sets three fasting days for every week; and 6:1 diet which only involves one fasting day in a week. If you don't find yourself fit to practice fasting for two days every week, then you can try some of these variations. As long as you stick to cutting your calorie intake into 25% during fasting periods, there shouldn't be any problem.

Eat-Stop-Eat Diet Plan

The eat-stop-eat diet plan was created by weight-loss expert Brad Pilon based on the concept of intermittent fasting. Pilon has a background in sports nutrition and supplements that is why this specific diet plan, according to diet experts, is more suitable for people who are usually involved in physical activities or sports.

In an eat-stop-eat diet plan, you fast for full 24 hours once or twice a week; thus, it is also called the 24-hour fast plan. Similar to 5:2 diet, you may eat normally during your non-fasting days. However, if both the consecutive and non-consecutive fast days are acceptable in 5:2 diet, in eat-stop-eat diet plan, only the non-consecutive days are deemed appropriate. In fact, Pilon even expressly emphasized that one should not fast for consecutive days and neither should one fast for more than 48 hours in a single week.

There are no quantified calorie limits during fast days in this type of intermittent fasting; as you should aim for a complete abstinence from food if you are following eat-stop-eat diet. You can, however, take diet soda, sparkling water, tea, or coffee during such period. If you felt the need to break the full fast, Pilon says that you can eat whatever you want to eat but he also suggests that you moderate your consumption. Also, if you cannot fast for 24 hours straight, shorter periods will also work as long as it is not less than 20 hours.

After the 24-hour fast, it is advised that appropriate amount of calorie intake per day should be taken— approximately 2000 calories for women and 2500 calories for men. Also, high-quality protein is highly recommended in this diet. You may take 20 to 30 grams of it every four to five hours for a total of 100 grams per day. This is to ensure that lean muscle mass is retained during intermittent fasting.

Say, if you started your fast at 8 am on Tuesday, you can resume eating normally at 8 am on Wednesday. During the fasting period, starting at 8 am on Tuesday, you may drink coffee or diet soda and consume a total of 100 grams of high-quality protein. If you still find it hard to go through the day without eating meals, you may eat a little but make sure to limit it otherwise it cannot be considered as a fasting period. You can have your breakfast exactly at 8 am in the next morning as the fasting period ends at that time. You can go back to eating normally and after several non-fasting days, you can then repeat the 24-hour fast.

Remember, your fasting days should not be near to each other for this kind of plan not only is after weight loss but is also aiming to maintain lean muscle mass. Pilon also does not recommend pairing this diet schedule with low-carb meals as this will only result into energy deficiency. Individuals who adopt this type of intermittent fasting need appropriate levels of energy; hence, appropriate amount of glucose. This is also the reason that Pilon recommends taking the right amount of calorie intake per non-fasting day. The results of this diet plan are enhanced by consumption of fruits and vegetables.

16:8 Protocol

This intermittent fasting variant was originated by

personal trainer and nutritional expert Martin Ber-khan. Unlike the first two mentioned diet plans, this is a day-based fasting; which means that a cycle takes only a day to repeat and that each day is split into fasting and eating hours. 16:8 simply means a day should be composed of 16 hours of fasting and 8 hours of free-eating. The diet plan is known for its effectiveness not only to weight loss but also to lean mass gain, that's why Berkhan calls it the "leangains" method. You'll find out more about this type of inter-mittent fasting on the part II of this book.

The Warrior Diet

Ever imagined a Viking devouring a whole table of foods? What about a Spartan gulping a big barrel of wine? Well, one of these days, you might find your-self looking like these men as you take your meal un-der the Warrior Diet plan.

The Warrior Diet is one of the most popular diet plans that incorporate intermittent fasting. There is actually a whole book discussing about this and it was written by nutritional and fitness expert Ori Hof-mekler, who apparently started this kind of diet philosophy. Hofmekler is the founder of Defense Nutrition. He has already authored a number of books to date, all of which tackle health and fitness.

So, how is Warrior Diet done? The diet plan essentially follows a day-based intermittent fasting schedule. On each day, you have to fast for 20 hours straight and eat at least once during the remaining four hours. The fasting period of 20 hours might sound like an uphill battle to some, considering it must be applied every—single—day; but don't worry, the fasting period in this diet protocol allows consumption of minimal servings of raw fruits and veggies, or a glass of fresh juice. You may also take small servings of protein if you want. Just don't eat a full-course meal during fast.

Fasting and eating periods under this diet pattern are more appropriately termed as "undereating" and "overeating" periods, respectively. So, we can say that the undereating phase is really intended for you to still be able to consume foods although such consumption must strictly be observed and limited. Overeating phase, on the other hand, is the four-hour period where you can eat tons of foods covering as many nutrients as possible. It is also important to set the overeating phase at night time.

For example, if you choose to set your overeating phase at six o'clock to ten o'clock in the evening, you must limit your food intake from 10 pm of the same night to 6 pm of the next day. During your 20-hour undereating phase you may take a small plate of pure vegetable salad or drink freshly extracted fruit or vegetable juice. You can also add a bit of protein to your salad by putting a few strips of lean chicken meat to it. Once the clock turns to 6 pm, you can now "overeat" as pointedly instructed by the diet plan. You may eat a large meal composed of a bowl of Caesar salad, a plate of steak and seared salmon, as well as a dish of carbonara or a clubhouse sandwich if you want to. Yes, this diet plan does mean it when it says to eat "tons" of foods. Besides, it isn't called Warrior Diet for nothing.

Speaking of being a "warrior" in this diet plan, you also need to discipline yourself like one. The diet protocol does not just instruct eating a lot during the four-hour overeating phase, it also highly recommends proper sequence of food intake once you start with your free-eating period. The order of food intake from first to last should be: vegetables, protein, fat, and carbohydrates. The first three should as much as possible be strictly taken in order. You may omit the carbohydrates if you want but you'd most likely need to eat some, considering this comes after a long period of fasting. The carbs are neither limited anyway so you can take as much as you want as long as they come after the veggies, protein, and fat.

The science behind this diet plan is a bit complex to explain. Contrary to the common diet rule that one should not eat late at night, as such will only result to weight gain, the philosophy that backs up this diet plan is linked to a different theory—humans are inherently nocturnal eaters. But despite holding on to a different view, nutrition experts are convinced with the protocol's effects in the body.

To explain, the undereating phase is meant to maximize "fight or flight" response of the sympathetic nervous system. Fight-or-flight response is a reaction made by the body in response to a perceived threat. Threat includes harmful events, imminent danger, or even survival threats like hunger. And since the body struggles with hunger during the 20-hour fast, the fight-or-flight responds by making the body more alert and boosting the energy which would eventually result to stimulating the fat burning process.

The overeating phase, on the other hand, is supposed to utilize the ability of the Parasympathetic Nervous System to promote digestion, as well as relaxation within the body. This allows the body to absorb the consumed nutrients and use it for repair and growth. It also helps the body burn fats during the day.

The benefits of Warrior Diet to the body will only be maximized if one follows the plan accordingly. Majority of those who tried this diet plan claim that this is a tough job to take. But at the end of the day, being able to witness the progress in your body is what matters the most. After all, it's a diet plan for the devoted and disciplined individuals—for the warriors-in-training.

Alternate-Day Fasting

Alternate-day fasting or up-day-down-day diet is a fasting protocol that follows a two-day cycle. It originated from the book UpDayDownDay Diet™ which was authored by plastic surgeon Dr. James Johnson.

Doctor Johnson also struggled with weight loss himself, which led him to the discovery of an eating plan effective for weight loss.

The diet plan is fairly plain; you eat minimal servings of meals one day and you eat your usual servings the next day. In here, the days when you eat small or limited servings are called "down days" while those which allow you to consume normal servings are called "up days." The process simply repeats every two days and since it's a two-day cycle, there are really no particular days which can be set as either up days or down days (if your Monday this week is a down day then your Monday next week won't be the same assuming you followed the fasting schedule throughout the week).

The plan also entails a quantified limit of calorie intake that should be followed on down days as much as possible. It instructs that you only consume one fifth of your usual calorie intake during your down days. Therefore, if your normal consumption is approximately 2000 calories per day, then you should only take approximately 400 calories on your down days. Your down days would typically comprise regular or normal meals although those must come in smaller servings.

According to Doctor Johnson, if you find it hard to stick to your down days, you may opt for protein and calorie shakes or meal replacement shakes. These shakes are packed with essential nutrients and can safely substitute meals. However, these shakes are merely a help for you to survive down days especially when you are a beginner to this. They should only be taken on your first two weeks under this diet schedule and should not be a regular substitute for your meals every down day. After at most, two weeks, you should go back to eating "real" foods or meals so your body won't get used to depending on liquids and shakes.

If you are a gym rat, you might want to consider hitting the gym only on your up days, as these are the days on which you can surely sustain endurance on physical activities without breaking the diet plan. Lifting weights and engaging to other strenuous activities require quite a pack of energy and you can only have a decent amount of it on days when you eat "normal" or "enough" servings. Besides, alternate-day fasting is designed solely to promote weight loss.

Trying to gain lean muscle mass while under this diet plan would entail additional efforts and those include disciplining your gym-enthusiast-self to rest on down days (and probably to eat more protein-rich servings).

Fat Loss Forever

If you're torn between the flexibility of eat-stop-eat diet and the free-eating feature of Warrior Diet, Fat Loss Forever diet might be the one that you're looking for. The diet plan was conceptualized by fitness expert John Romaniello and was made for gym-goers who want a flexible diet schedule that also includes the most important day of the week—cheat day.

The name "Fat Loss Forever" is actually a fancy title for a diet plan with a complicated mixture of different fasting protocols in one schedule. Unless you pull off the diet schedule properly, the "fat loss" is not going to come and the possibility that the fat will be lost "forever" won't be guaranteed. Nevertheless, it's still labeled as one of the most effective diet plans anchored to the concept of intermittent fasting.

The diet plan is essentially a week-based intermittent fasting and each week should include two primary periods: the cheat day and the 36-hour fast. The 36-hour fast should always come after the cheat day. After that, you should incorporate one or more intermittent fasting protocols for the rest of the week. Romaniello suggests that you save your 36-hour fast for the busiest days of your week so you'd be focused on more important things (e.g. work) other than your hunger.

Let's say, if you started your cheat day on Thursday at 8 am and ate your last "cheat" meal for the day at 9 pm, your 36-hour fast should start at 9 pm on the same day. Counting 36 hours from 9 pm, your next "normal meal" should be on Saturday at 9 am. That is indeed a long period of fast but of course, you can consume small servings of protein, carbs, fruits, and vegetables during the 36-hour period; just make sure you are not taking any full-course meal. Afterwards, if you decided to adopt alternate-day fasting for the rest of the week, then the day after your 36-hour fast (Saturday in this case) should be an up day as your body needs to recover enough nutrients after the fast. The next day which is Sunday, should then be a down day. The remaining days before the next Thursday should just be an alternating series of up and down days.

It is important to apply the corresponding rules under the different fasting protocols that you use for the rest of the week, after the cheat day and 36-hour fast. From the illustration above, your down days should only comprise one fifth of your average calorie consumption. If you happen to consume an average of approximately 2500 calories a day, you should limit your Sunday and Tuesday meals at 500 calories (one fifth of 2500) for the whole day.

For another example, let's say you started your cheat day on Sunday from 9 am to 10 pm. This sets your 36-hour fasting period at 10 pm on Sunday and from that, the period should end at 10 am on Tuesday. If you use the Warrior Diet for the rest of the week, then that forces you to extend the 36-hour fasting period to 44 to 48 hours. This is because the Warrior Diet follows a night-time eating schedule; and since your 36-hour fasting period ends at morning, you'll need to wait for another couple of hours before you can eat. Therefore, your next large meal should be on Tuesday around 6 or 8 pm. For Wednesday up to Saturday, the night-time eating rule shall also be applied accordingly. You can have your cheat day once again when the next Sunday arrives.

With regard to cheat days, it is crucial that you know what to eat when you are given such heavenly freedom. On these days, cakes, ice cream, sodas, fast foods, junk foods, or charred meats might be enticing but are they really worth it? Well, considering that you sacrificed probably the majority of your week in the name of fasting, those are more or less fine to eat (it's a cheat day anyway). You deserve them!

However, it will be a lot better if you focus on eating the healthier foods which offer all the nutrients that you were deprived of during the past few days of struggle. You fasted, so you technically did not just lose fats; some essential nutrients were also lost along the way. At least try to eat a lot of vegetables, fruits, lean meats, and healthy amount of fats and carbs first before taking the not-so-healthy second options. Also, do not forget the fact that anything taken excessively has corresponding undesirable effects.

The diet might seem so complicated at first but once you and your body get used to it, you'll find out that it's actually a rewarding diet plan. Plus, your body will also be able to flexibly adapt to changes as you switch from one diet protocol to another in order to fit in with your ever-changing personal schedule. Just stick to the two important parts of the week namely, the cheat day and the 36-hour fasting period; and let the rest of the week adapt to whatever intermittent fasting plans you decide to use.

PART II – COMPREHENSIVE GUIDE TO INTERMITTENT FASTING

CHAPTER 6

TAKING THE ACTION

If you already feel, by now, that you're ready to take the action and start implementing intermittent fasting to your daily life, you might want to consider to take it easy. Not that being excited is bad, though. It's just that, this is one of those points in your life when you should stop your happily excited spirit from rushing things out. Why?

A lot of people fail to realize that just because you have already learned the basics and foundational concepts of intermittent fasting, doesn't mean you are fully ready to apply it in your life. Those who failed with their diet plans most probably overlooked something that could've otherwise made their weight-loss journey successful—preparation.

Reading about fasting is different from actually doing it. It's easier said than done. Therefore, preparation must come in between reading and practicing. And to help you with your preparation, you may consider the following order of guidelines: self-assessment, choosing a diet plan, understanding the importance of exercise, and learning about the fasting foods and liquids.

Assessing Yourself

First things first—are you ready? In intermittent fasting, being ready doesn't just refer to your body's capability to undergo sets of fasting periods; it also refers to your mental state of readiness. Being physically ready to intermittent fasting is generally easy. The human body can inherently last even up to two weeks without food. So, the real question would be, are you mentally ready?

You need to assess yourself as early as now because if you are not mentally ready, chances are you'll end up breaking your fasting rules, ditching your fasting periods, disregarding your diet, giving in to temptations, or worse, losing your motivation halfway. The reason you need to assess yourself is that you'll be sacrificing time and effort for this matter, and you probably wouldn't want to spend significant amounts of these two precious things just to find out that you don't want to continue with your diet plan anymore.

If you are, however, sure that you are ready for a change in your lifestyle and that you can take or endure whatever it may bring, then you can expect that everything else that follows after this first stage of preparation would be easy for you.

Choosing a Diet Plan

The worst part about choosing a diet plan, most especially if you are a beginner, is that you are not sure whether your chosen plan will be successful or not; and that it takes at least a month before you can say if you made the right choice or not. The truth is, each and every type of intermittent fasting diet plan entails a risk of failure and that there's no such thing as a "perfect" diet plan that can absolutely guarantee either weight loss or muscle mass gain, not even among the most prominent ones listed in the previous chapter.

There is, however, a measure that can help you minimize the risk of failing with a diet program; we'll call it personal filtering. Personal filtering simply means that you filter out, among the options you have, the one which best suits your preferences. It's a pre-implementation analysis that identifies which among the option, prior to its implementation, could provide the most positive outcome by examining the features of each available option. The main idea is to remove as many options as possible from the choices you have until you come up with, most preferably, one option which will then be deemed as fit for you.

To demonstrate, let's try to use the types of intermittent fasting given in the previous chapter (except for the 16:8 protocol since it was not yet discussed thoroughly). The first eliminating question should be, "what is your goal?" Are you after weight loss? Muscle gain? Or both? Assuming you are after both, then that already removes Fat Loss Forever Diet from the list since it's designed solely for weight loss. Next question would be, "how much fasting can you endure?" The question can be answered as a number of hours per day or a number of days per week. Suppose that your work schedule only permits fasting for a maximum of two days a week. This cancels out The Warrior Diet and the Alternate-day fasting from your choices as both require more than two days of fasting in a single week.

You now have narrowed down your choices into two: the 5:2 diet and the Eat-Stop-Eat diet. The deciding factor should now be based on the differences between the two. The 5:2 diet is a more flexible than Eat-Stop-Eat as you can fast for either two straight consecutive days or two non-consecutive days. It is also good if you only want to limit your consumption during fasting days rather than to completely abstain from it. Plus, it goes with a quantified limit (25% of your average daily calorie intake) so in case you feel like you're going beyond limit you can just check it through computation.

Eat-stop-eat on the other hand, best suits the sports and gym enthusiasts as such diet plan is specifically made for them. If you are seriously devoted to fasting, this is also a better choice since the goal in each fasting day is full abstinence. Now, assuming you are a sports enthusiast whose desire to lose weight and gain muscle mass is at peak, then your final choice would obviously be the Eat-stop-eat Diet.

It is important to remember that personal filtering is merely a guide to help you choose the most appropriate diet plan for you. It does not guarantee success although it can be inferred that it somehow increases your chance to succeed since through it, you'll be able to choose the diet program which can be implemented in accordance to your schedule and needs.

Recognizing Exercise as an Important Factor to Weight Loss

If your ultimate goal for using intermittent fasting is to shed pounds, then from now on, you must see weight-loss exercises as your biggest friend. It is true that intermittent fasting alone can burn your fats and provide evident results; but pairing it with proper exercise, you'll cut the progress time almost into half. Yes, with proper guidance and consistent dedication, these rather exhausting activities could accelerate the results.

Of course, if you are new to diet plans and intermittent fasting, you do not have to engage immediately on physical exercise. Let your body adapt to the changes first and when you feel like it already has, you can start by choosing which set of exercises is suitable for your physique, for your endurance, and most importantly, for your diet program.

Learning About Fasting Foods and Liquids

Pre-familiarizing yourself with the foods and drinks you can take during partially restricted fasting periods is also important. It's because most of the diet plans under intermittent fasting allow consumption of minimal servings of foods during fast hours or days. In general, foods that are considered safe during fasts include vegetables and fruits, whole grains, low-fat and low-sodium foods.

Liquids on the other hand are usually more available and safer during fasts. Water and fresh juices are typically recommended when you are under intermittent fasting. Protein or meal replacement shakes are also used in some techniques. Smoothies, juices, and shakes that are made up of nutrients-rich ingredients are also advised to be taken.

If you want to know the particular options you have, there is a list provided on the latter part of the book that enumerates specific fasting foods and liquids you can take during partially restricted fasting periods.

It must be emphasized that the measures above are mere guidelines for you to maximize the potential results of any weight-loss program that you decide to implement in your lifestyle. They do not guarantee perfect outcomes. The only key to make sure that a diet plan is going to provide desirable results is strict adherence. Honestly, all of these diet plans are programmed to work but unless you follow them correctly, you can never achieve optimum results. Temptations and frustrations already await you the moment you take your first step to your weight-loss journey. So, let me ask you the question once again— are you ready?

CHAPTER 7

THE BEGINNER'S PROTOCOL

By now you should have assessed yourself and have also decided that you are going to openly welcome intermittent fasting to your life—that's the spirit! And assuming you are indeed done with the self-assessment process, let's now proceed to the second step which is choosing the best type of intermittent fasting-based diet plan.

Whether you are new exclusively to intermittent fasting or completely new to diet plans in general, there's one type of intermittent fasting that would likely fit your current lifestyle, and would only incur little changes in your daily life once implemented. If you are, however, neither of the two, don't worry because this diet plan is also suitable to everyone else, even if you are a healthy person of normal weight. The diet plan is called the 16:8 method.

16:8 Method - How It Is Done

As once explained in chapter 5, this diet plan was introduced by personal trainer and nutritional expert Martin Berkhan. It's a daily intermittent fasting which divides each day into 16 hours of fasting period and 8 hours of normal- or free-eating period. The original term for this method was "Leangains method" as referred to by Berkhan but the term "16:8 method" is kind of getting more and more popular than the former. In this book, we'll also refer to it as the beginner's protocol.

The first thing to consider in 16:8 protocol is on which part of the day should both the fasting and eating periods be set. Fortunately, there exists a "standard" setting for both periods so you might want to just adopt it since it has already been tested and proven by the majority of 16:8 diet plan followers. Under the said setting, the 16-hour fasting period runs from 8 pm one day to 12 pm or 12 noon the next day. This means that, in a single day, you can only eat from 12 pm to 8 pm.

Such standardized setting is not really that hard to implement. Come to think of it, a dinner at let's say, 7:30 pm is quite an appropriate time considering that you are most probably in a fat-loss diet. It's not too early which means your body can sustain hunger before sleeping time; and neither is it too late which means proper digestion can still be expected.

There are no restrictions with regard to the meals that you can take during the eight-hour eating window; thus, you can eat normal meals at normal servings. Most of the people who practice the 16:8 method, however, cuts the number of meals they take into two. They usually skip breakfast since the eating window starts at lunch time anyway. Nonetheless, you can still stick to taking three regular-sized meals a day if you want to, as long as you take all three within the eating window.

The schedule simply repeats every day. You can expect your first few days or weeks to be burdensome but once your body adapts to the cycle, you'll get used to it and most importantly, you'll start to notice the progress.

Benefits of 16:8 Method

- Increased Chances of Fat Loss

  Since your body's metabolism becomes slower as it enters the sleeping state, it naturally functions slower at night. Therefore, anything that is consumed beyond 8 pm to 9 pm, or at any time near bed time, won't likely be burned properly. This is the reason 16:8 method is a top choice when it comes to weight loss. It limits the chances of calories getting stored as fats by setting the dinner or last meal for the day, at an earlier and safer hour. And because the body is most probably secured from obtaining unwanted increase in fat mass, it'll be easier to lose weight.

- Lean Mass Retention

  The body weight comprises two major composition namely, fat mass and lean mass. Therefore, when we say "weight loss," it can refer to the loss of either fat mass or lean mass; but most of the time, both. The ideal result, however, is to lose fat mass but not lean mass. Lean mass is important as it includes muscle mass which certainly needs to be maintained as much as possible, to keep your muscle strength at an optimal level. Fortunately, 16:8 method promotes retention of much of the lean mass in the body amid significant reduction in fat mass.

- Controlled Hunger

In 16:8 diet plan, your eating window is narrowed down to an eight-hour period. This eventually leads to changes in your body's natural cravings. Of course, you won't notice the effect on your first few weeks under the diet plan; but if you continue to commit yourself to the plan, your body will start to "reprogram" itself and get used to not feeling much of the usual, stubbornly constant hunger. Plus, it'll also be easier for you to get satisfied with meals.

- Improved Insulin Response

An improved insulin response is a contributory factor to both the lean mass retention and the controlled hunger mentioned above. But aside from that, it also makes insulin levels more stable that's why some of the people who are at risk of diabetes type 2 devotedly follow 16:8 method.

- Enhanced Brain Function

  If you're stressing about not being able to think properly while fasted, then let 16:8 method cut your worries. On your first few days under 16:8 method, your brain will probably not function well as it's still trying to adapt to certain changes. But once it has, you'll notice that your mentality can function just as normally as it could before intermittent fasting—or even better. This is because your body is not forced to pump large amount of blood to your digestive system when you are fasted. Thus, it's able to deliver more oxygen to other parts including your brain.

Constructing Your Own 16:8 Schedule

For most people, especially to beginners, it's highly advised to implement 16:8 diet using the standard, 12 pm to 8 pm eating-window schedule. However, if your personal schedule does not permit such setting or you simply don't want to follow the norm, then you can schedule your own plan to fit your lifestyle.

The first question to ask here is which among the three major meals is going to be eliminated? The answer will either be based on your schedule or be coming from your own preference although you should also consider the importance of each meal to your weight-loss goal. Putting that in mind, it would be best for you to skip dinner. If it's impossible, however, your second-best choice would be eliminating breakfast so as to make sure that any excess on your dinner intake still has time to be burned in the morning. Lunch is the most unlikely to be eliminated since the meals that you consume on your lunch time are more or less burned properly regardless if you are under a diet plan or not.

Say, for example, your work starts at 8 am and ends at 3 pm, your best option would be skipping dinner, as it is the time of the day when much, if not all, of your work is probably done; hence, no hunger-triggering activity. Skipping breakfast might be dangerous when you are a complete beginner to fasting. So, for such situation, you may start your eating window at 7:30 am to 3:30 pm. Within such window, you can eat your breakfast at 7:30 am or 7:45 am, before you go to work; and have your last meal right exactly at 3 pm, after work or a little later at 3:30 pm. Addition of an in-between meal is not much of an issue here so you can have lunch at 11 am or 12 pm and still eat some more after work as long as it's covered by the eating window.

If you can, however, endure a no-breakfast morning even at work, you can move the beginning of your eating window to 11 am to 12 pm or exactly to your lunch break. If your lunch break starts at 11 am, then you can eat your lunch at 11 am and adjust your last meal time to 7 pm, or to any time earlier than that. If you get used to this setting, you'll find out that it's actually easier and better to skip breakfast as you can expect an increase in focus and other brain functions as previously explained in the benefits of 16:8 method.

Your eating-window also does not necessarily have to be a full eight-hour period. You may further narrow it down into seven or four hours. However, such is only advisable if you have been using intermittent fasting for a long period of time. If you are still beginning to adapt to the lifestyle, then sticking to an eight-hour eating window is strongly recommended.

Cheat Days - to Cheat or Not to Cheat?

16:8 method is not a religious devotion so you can start celebrating because apparently, cheat day is allowed under this diet schedule. Some of the followers of the diet plan claimed that they've still succeeded losing significant weight even if they admittedly cheated for a couple of days in some of the weeks. The safest number of cheat days you can have per week is one; but it's not a hard and fast rule so you can have your cheat days for two or three days a week. Just make sure that majority of the days in your week still follow the 16:8 plan, especially if you really are into achieving weight loss.

Also, it would be better not to overeat on your cheat days. A cheat day only means that you can extend your eating-window for more than eight hours or you can simply break the fasting period; but it does not mean that you should eat a lot of sweets and fatty foods every hour. Always eat in moderation whether it involves a healthy or unhealthy food. The result of 16:8 diet plan largely depends on you so always consider that.

Famous People with 16/8-Diet-Bodies

Actor Hugh Jackman, majorly known for playing the role of Wolverine in the X-men movies, is one of the most prominent Hollywood figures to date. The actor has always been a center of interest to diet experts and fitness magazines for his ripped, Wolverine physique which Jackman proudly claims to be the result of his 16:8 diet schedule. At least now you know that the secret to Wolverine's size and strength is not found on his mutant genes—but to 16:8 diet.

Another popular actor who uses 16:8 diet plan is Terry Crews. He explained that his eating-window goes from 2 pm to 10 pm and he fasts for the rest of the day. He also does not eat foods, even minimal amounts of it during fasts, although he drinks coffee or tea during such periods. According to Crews, the only problem with 16:8 method is that you don't want a "bad meal" for your eating period because no one waits for 16 hours just to end up eating a bad meal.

David Kingsburry, trainer of some celebrities including Chris Hemsworth, Michael Fassbender, and Jennifer Lawrence, also promotes the 16:8 diet plan because aside from its effectiveness, the schedule, as

Kingsburry said, can easily fit in an individual's life-style.

CHAPTER 8

THE COMPLEMENTARY GUIDE

After choosing the intermittent fasting diet plan, the guidelines state that the next two things to consider would be: learning about exercise and getting familiar with fasting foods and liquids. The first thing you need to know about these two is that they are both supplemental factors to intermittent fasting and are meant to help you maximize results.

Guide to Exercises

What's better than acquiring the weight-loss benefit of the beginner's protocol is maximizing the lean mass retention it features. It would be easier to gain muscle mass while under the diet plan since, as once mentioned earlier, much of the lean mass is retained despite weight loss. But if you are only after the weight loss, then that's equally fine. In any case, it's important that you utilize your 16-hour fasting window for many positive things can happen within that period of time.

The ideal time to apply weight-loss exercises while under intermittent fasting would be during the fasted period, most preferably in the morning. Considering you skip breakfasts during your 16-hour fasts, a complete exercise in the morning can burn significant amount of fats in your body. Provided below is a list of some of the well-known exercises that you may do every morning, to help accelerate the fat burning process and maintain your weight-loss progress:

- Squats

- Lunges (including explosive lunges)

- Kettlebell Swings

- Tabata Drill

- Double Jump

- Body-Weight Exercises

- Burpees

- Mountain Climbers

- Jump Rope

Guide to Training and Workout

Guidelines for strength training and muscle workouts are essentially stricter than weight-loss exercises. This is because in the latter, the only goal is to lose weight while in the former, the objective is to gain muscle mass while losing weight at the same time.

Training or workout may be done either during a fasted period or within an eating window. If you cannot commit to a fasted training, then it would be more appropriate if you train or work out in the middle of your eating window. In such case, you have to secure three meals within your eating window to support your system.

To illustrate, assume for example that you adopted the standard 16:8 schedule. This means that your workout shall be within the eating window, 12 pm to 8 pm. Your 12-noon lunch shall serve as your pre-workout meal. It must comprise 20-25% of your daily calorie intake. After that, your training should be set around 3:30 to 4:00 pm (it is important that the training is set at least an hour after pre-workout meal). Assuming the training takes an hour, your post-workout meal should be around 4:30 to 5:00 pm. Your post-workout meal should always be the largest meal. You should then take your dinner or the last meal of the day at either 7:00 pm or 8:00 pm to help you sustain the following fasting period.

It is also possible that you take two pre-workout meals before working out. Let's use one of the examples we had last chapter (eating window at 7:30 am to 3:30 pm) for demonstration. Your breakfast at 7:30 am should serve as your first pre-workout meal. Your next meal, let's say at 11:30 am, should then be your second pre-workout meal. Each of your pre-workout meals should consist 20-25% of your daily calorie consumption. Counting a few hours from your second pre-workout meal, you may start your training at 2:30 pm. Assuming again that your training takes only an hour, your post-workout, and last meal for the day should be taken exactly at 3:30 pm.

Now for the fasted training, you should first familiarize yourself with the branched-chain amino acids or BCAAs. These are amino acids usually taken, in the form of tablets or powder, to stimulate protein synthesis especially during trainings or workouts. Protein synthesis is essential for muscle growth and stimulating it serves as a defense against protein breakdown.

For a workout day, it is strongly recommended that you ready three 10-gram BCAA tablets or a 30-gram BCAA powder. The BCAA supplements will be used throughout a portion your fasted period. You should take one 10-gram BCAA tablet after your pre-workout. Afterward, you can proceed to your workout. Take another tablet an hour after your workout and take the last one two hours after your last intake. If you are going to use the powder, simply mix it in a shake or in a drink and divide the whole drink into three equal servings.

To demonstrate using the standard schedule, if you wake up at 6 am, your first tablet shall be taken after a five- to fifteen-minute pre-workout. Your training shall then start at 7 am and end at 8 am assuming it's a one-hour training. You shall take the second tablet around 8 am, right after the training. The last tablet shall then be taken at 10 am, two hours after the last intake.

Your lunch at 12 pm should serve as your post-workout meal; hence, the largest meal of the day. Your dinner or last meal should normally be taken at 8 pm. It's up to you if you want to consume in-between meals. If you commit to this strategy, your body will gain more muscle strength and will only lose fat mass in the process.

Guide to 16:8 Diet-Specific Fasting Foods and Liquids

There are no fasting foods that are labeled safe to be consumed during the 16-hour period. To be honest, the fasting period in beginner's protocol is not much of a burden if you compare it to other fasting periods; like the 20-hour fast in Warrior Diet or the two-day fast under 5:2 Diet. Therefore, fasting foods aren't really an ultimate necessity. And the only means available to ease your 16-hour struggle are gums and fasting liquids.

Gums are good for people who often confuse boredom with hunger. If you're bored and you feel like the only answer to it is food, then try chewing a gum. Sometimes, you're not really craving for a food but instead, you just want to chew something in your mouth. The gum, however, that is referred to in this guide is a sugar-free gum. Sweeteners on regular chewing gums will only break your fast so you should avoid them.

In terms of fasting liquids, you can drink water if you want. As a matter of fact, you should drink a lot of it during fast. It does not only improve your metabolism but it also helps suppress hunger. Detox water, is also counted and is actually more preferable. Try adding a mint leaf or a slice of lemon to each glass to obtain better and more refreshing effects.

Black coffee and green tea can also save you from your fasting struggles most especially during the morning. They can help increase fat burning process and delay hunger. These beverages, however, should not come with large amounts of milk and sugar.

Take note that all of these are specifically applicable only to 16:8 diet protocol. Some diet plans do not allow most or all of the foods and drinks stated above, while some allow a wider range of options. If you want to learn more about the general fasting foods and liquids that are allowed under most of intermittent fasting-based diet plans, you can check the list provided in the next chapter.

PART III - SUPPLEMENTAL SECTION

CHAPTER 9

FASTING FOODS AND
LIQUIDS

Contrary to the traditional fasting that refers to absolute abstinence from foods and liquids, intermittent
fasting refers to a period where one's consumption is
limited only to some fasting specifications. The limits
among diet plans slightly vary depending on which
type of intermittent fasting you opted to follow. Nevertheless, there are specific foods and liquids that are
generally present and allowed in almost any type of
diet plan.

Fruits and Vegetables

The tandem always tops almost any list of ideal foods
that must be eaten for a healthier life. This is obviously because fruits and vegetables are legitimate

sources of vitamins and minerals. Plus, they are naturally high in antioxidants. You can eat a serving or two of either a fruit salad or vegetable salad during your partially restricted fasting period. Or you can just directly eat a raw fruit or veggie for convenience. Below is a list of the most recommended fruits that you may consume during fasted periods:

- Green Apples

- Strawberries

- Oranges

- Blackberries

- Cranberries

- Grapefruit

- Papaya

- Cantaloupes

- Raisins

- Apricots

- Guava

Roughly speaking, any vegetable, as long as it's not canned, is fairly good during fasted periods. However, there are vegetables which pack a particular combination of nutrients fit for an empty stomach; hence, perfect for fasting periods. Some of these vegetables are:

- Spinach

- Mustard Greens

- Cauliflower

- Brussels Sprouts

- Tomatoes

- Kale

- Lettuce

- Broccoli

- Cabbage

- Bok Choy

- Swiss Chard

Take note that the available fruits and vegetables appropriate for your fasting periods are not limited to the lists given above. Those just list the most recommended ones as they contain the vitamins and minerals that your body specially needs during fasted state. You have several more choices beyond those included in the list.

Nuts

In some intermittent fasting variants, foods which contain fats are allowed, and even suggested, to be consumed during fasted periods. So, to ensure that you are getting only the healthy fats, you can opt to go with nuts. Nuts contain both monounsaturated and polyunsaturated fats. These fats are also known as the good fats.

Good fats are "good" because they help lower your risk of stroke and other heart diseases and they also help lower cholesterol levels. Furthermore, they also contain omega-3 fatty acids, fiber, L-arginine, and vitamin E, all of which are known for being heart-friendly substances. The healthiest nuts that you can eat during fasting period are listed below:

- Brazil Nuts

- Macadamia Nuts

- Cashews

- Pecans

- Pine Nuts

- Walnuts

- Almonds

- Chestnuts

- Pistachios

Of course, nuts during fasting periods should be limited accordingly to what your specific diet plan allows. The main reason they are fine to eat during fasted state is that they satisfy the body almost the same way as meats do. Therefore, they can somehow extend your body's endurance to hunger. Their benefits, especially to the heart, are also considered as a contributory factor.

Soups

If you want to spend your fasted period eating something with a meaty taste but your diet plan only allows liquid, then the best option you have is a soup. Soups are easily digested by the body so it can be safely taken without worrying about breaking the fast. The ideal number of servings for a soup during a fasted period is one; but taking two bowls of it won't hurt your fasting. Try to limit soup intake only up to two servings per fasting period. To name a few diet-friendly soups, we have:

- Vegetable Broth

- Spinach-Artichoke Soup

- Moroccan Stew

- Corn Chowder

- Black Bean Minestrone

- Lentil-Vegetable Soup

- Carrot and Ginger Soup

Protein and Meal Replacement Shakes

First on the list of fasting liquids are the protein and meal replacement shakes. Protein shakes are flavored shakes which contain large amounts of protein good for working out and training. Meal replacement shakes, on the other hand, contain almost similar substances except that they have lower protein content, but higher calorie content than protein shakes.

If the fasting periods under your specific diet plan limit meals into a certain number of calories per day, it will be best for you to substitute your meal with a meal replacement shake. Meal replacement shakes have quantifiable calorie amounts (e.g. 400 calories per glass) so it will be easier for you to track your calorie intake during fasted periods.

If you are more into training during your fasted days, going for protein shakes is a wise idea. A protein shake, with its massive protein content, can help support your muscle strength throughout and after training. Plus, measuring calorie intake with protein shakes is easy as well.

Detox Water

You can safely drink a detox water under any inter-mittent fasting plan. Detox water is simply a plain wa-ter with a bit of "detoxifying" agents in it, like mint leaves, orange slices, or cinnamon sticks. And since it combines the cleansing-benefit of water and the fat-burning, detoxifying properties of herbs or fruits, into one glass, it's pretty much a better option to drink than plain drinking water. You get to be cleansed and detoxified at the same time.

Fresh Juices and Smoothies

Making a smoothie or juice out of fruits or vegetables is a common practice among people who couldn't stand a fasting period without sipping a refreshing flavored drink. There are no specifications about which flavors of juices and smoothies must be drunk. As long as a juice or smoothie is made from fresh, raw, and organic fruits and vegetables, a glass or two of the drink is perfectly fine.

Coffees and Teas

Teas are more flexible in fasting than coffees. You can

drink a cup of jasmine tea, green tea, or any tea during fasted periods. Teas contain few calories and they won't derail your fasting protocol. They can also be served either hot or cold but a hot tea is more preferred by most.

On the other hand, only black coffees are allowed during fasted periods. It is also advised not buy coffees from coffee shops, as they roughly contain excessive amount of artificial sweetener, and high-fat creamers. If you want to add some sugar to your tea or coffee, you may do so as long as you limit such at regulated amounts.

CHAPTER 10

RECIPES FOR THE HUNGRY

You, and everyone else who follow any type of intermittent fasting will always have something in common—you're all at your hungriest a few minutes before the eating window starts. And you know what's better than being able to eat after a long period of starvation? The foods, themselves.

Your first and last meals (or perhaps any meal within the eating window) are considerably precious to you that's why there's really no space for—as Terry Crews calls it—a "bad meal." So, consider rewarding yourself every time you survive a fasting period and serve some of the best recipes that you'll discover in this section.

Fresh Mexican Tuna Salad

It's a Pico de Gallo-inspired tuna recipe which combines protein-packed tuna with fresh veggies. It's low in fat and carbohydrates so you can eat more servings of this recipe during your eating window. It's a good post-workout meal too!

Ingredients:

- 2 large tomatoes (chopped)

- 1 large red onion (chopped)

- 1 bunch of Chinese parsley (chopped)

- 1 400-gram can of Tuna (flakes, preferably)

- 1 pc. of lime

Number of Servings:

2 bowls

Directions:

To get rid of the onions' aftertaste, place the chopped onion in a bowl and liberally sprinkle salt on it. Pour a cup of water into the bowl or until the salted onions are all covered with water. Let them sit for half an hour or until the onions have soaked. Afterwards, drain the onions and rinse with running water to remove any excess salt.

In a large bowl, mix the chopped tomatoes, Chinese parsley, and the onion. Squeeze a piece of lime over the mixture. Drain the can of tuna and combine the flakes with the vegetables. Gently toss the ingredients and serve.

Grilled BBQ Chicken Flatbreads

Eating pizza while under a diet plan might sound like an unforgivable sin—but if it's a pizza in the form of grilled flatbreads then it's totally fine. The recipe is an ideal snack to pack your calorie-deprived body with some calories and protein after a fasting period. Plus, this provides portion-controlled servings so there is nothing to worry about overeating.

<u>Ingredients:</u>

- 2 flatbreads

- 12 ounces chicken breast (boneless and skinless)

- 2 slices chopped Canadian bacon

- 1 cup of sliced red onions

- 1 cup of sliced bell pepper (yellow or red)

- 1 tbsp. fresh pineapple juice

- 1/4 cup chopped pineapple tidbits

- 1/4 cup barbeque sauce*

- 1/4 cup grated cheese

- a pinch of black pepper

Number of Servings:

4 slices

Directions:

Preheat the grill at 500 °F. On a grill tray, place the sliced onions and bell peppers then sprinkle on some pepper. Coat the chicken breast with cooking spray. Bring the chicken and the onions and bell peppers to grill. Cook each side of the chicken for three to four minutes or until the inside reaches 165 °F. Remove the veggies and chicken from the grill and then reduce the heat to 400 °F.

Transfer the chicken on to a cutting board and cut into strips or bite-sized pieces. In a blender, add the pineapple juice and barbecue sauce and pulse until the combination forms a thick sauce.

Place the flatbreads on a pizza stone or screen. Spread half a cup of the sauce on each flatbread, and top with the chicken cuts, Canadian bacon, grated cheese, grilled onions and bell peppers, and pineapple tid-bits; then place on the grill. Close the lid and wait for around 10 minutes to cook, or until the cheese has melted.

Remove from heat. Let the flatbread cool for a while before slicing; then serve.

Low-fat Chicken Spaghetti Carbonara

If you're a pasta lover then here's a simple recipe for you. This is specially made for people who devote themselves so much in a diet plan that they thought they are prohibited from indulging in dishes like Spaghetti Carbonara. But more importantly, this is made to complement low-fat diet plans.

Ingredients:

- 150 grams of pasta

- 1 skinless chicken breast (chopped)

- 4 short-cut lean bacon slices

- 2 cloves garlic (crushed)

- 1/2 onion (sliced)

- 2 spring onions (sliced)

- 1 tbsp. olive oil

- cracked pepper

- 3/4 cup light evaporative milk

2 plates

Directions:

Cook pasta as per instructions; then drain and set aside.

Preheat a non-stick fry-pan at medium heat. Add a little olive oil on the pan and cook bacon until crispy. Once the bacon becomes crispy, set it aside. Add a little olive oil again on the same pan then cook the onion on low heat until soft. Set the onion aside along with the bacon.

Add the remaining olive oil on the pan, turn to medium heat, and cook the chicken breast for around four to five minutes, until semi-cooked. Afterwards, slightly lower the heat and add the bacon and onion to the chicken, and then add garlic. Pour the evaporated milk then season with pepper to taste.

Stir the sauce occasionally while heating. Once the sauce bubbles, further lower the heat and add the cooked pasta. When the sauce turns into a slightly thick consistency, turn off the heat. Add the sliced spring onions then serve.

Green Tea Powerhouse Smoothie

There's no way that you won't look for a refreshing break after a heated struggle with your fasting period. And one of the best refreshments available for a conscious, weight-watcher is this antioxidant-rich smoothie recipe. Combine all the vitamins that your body would surely need after a fasting window and add a pack of protein to that—voila! A green tea powerhouse smoothie.

Ingredients:

- 1 bag of green tea

- ½ medium banana

- 1½ frozen blueberries

- ¾ light vanilla soy milk

- 3 tbsp. water

- 2 tsp. honey

Number of Servings:

1 glass

<u>Directions:</u>

Steam or microwave water in small bowl. Once steaming hot, add tea bag and let it brew for three to five minutes. Remove tea bag afterwards. Add honey and stir the mixture. In a blender, combine tea mixture, banana, blueberries, and soy milk. Blend on the highest setting. Transfer the smoothie into a glass and serve.

Protein-Packed Dark Choco-Almond Cookies

Dessert time is always more fun when you're not anxious about your weight and health. These cookies are going to bring your protein-diet gaming to the next level. Imagine being able to enjoy a delicious cookie while also gaining a dose of protein in every bite. It's a win-win situation, isn't it?

Ingredients:

- 1/4 cup unflavored protein powder

- 2 squares chopped dark chocolate (20 grams)

- 1/4 cup almonds (ground)

- 3 tbsp. almond butter

- 1/4 cup almond milk

- 1 tsp. coconut oil

- 2 tsp. coconut sugar

<u>Number of Servings:</u>

5 cookies

<u>Directions:</u>

Preheat oven to 350 °F. Mix protein powder, almonds, coconut sugar, almond butter, almond milk, and coconut oil together to make a dough. Once mixed, add dark chocolate. Roll dough into small-sized balls and place onto a tray lined with parchment paper. Flatten the balls with a spoon or with your fingers.

Place in the oven and bake for around 10 to 12 minutes or until baked. Remove from oven. Let the cookies rest to stiffen (and to prevent crumbling). Serve once completely cooled.

CONCLUSION

Perhaps, for the past centuries, people haven't found the ideal method of losing weight because we focused solely on the idea that what makes a person un-healthy or over-weight, is the kind of foods that he eats. Although it's legitimately true to some extent, it's not enough that we should focus only on a single idea and stop putting efforts to discover more from a different perspective.

Fortunately, intermittent fasting has been discovered right on the period when almost all of us are already giving up with our unsuccessful diet plans, brought by our desperate decisions—lots of thanks to the founders of the method!

And after reading all the chapters in this book, you have probably learned the important points about intermittent fasting. You discovered the method and learned about the science that, although is still being further proven by researchers across the globe, backs up much of the concept of the diet technique.

You also learned about the benefits of intermittent fasting not only to your weight but also to your overall health; from your insulin levels to your brain function. And above all, the method serves as a safer and even a better substitute to other diet plans as it has proven its purpose as a healthier way of losing weight and a bigger help to gaining muscle mass and strength.

You also know by now that there is a pool of options from which you can choose the type of intermittent fasting that best suits your lifestyle and needs. And if you can't decide on which among the options to choose, you can always go back to the book's comprehensive guide for beginners.

At this point, you already have everything you need to learn so you'd be able start your own journey to a healthy weight loss. Always remember that—regardless of the kind of diet plan that you implement, the outcome will always depend on your effort and most importantly, on your dedication. So, don't just do the process, commit yourself to it!

Thank you!

Before you go, I just wanted to say thank you for purchasing my book.

You could have picked from dozens of other books on the same topic but you took a chance and chose this one.

So, a HUGE thanks to you for getting this book and for reading all the way to the end.

Now I wanted to ask you for a small favor. **Could you please take just a few minutes to leave a review for this book on Amazon?**

This feedback will help me continue to write the type of books that will help you get the results you want. So if you enjoyed it, please let me know! (-:

Once again, don't forget to grab a copy of your FREE BONUS book "Super Foods For Super Health". If you are interested in learning more about the easily accessible super foods that you could incorporate into your diet and transform your overall health, then this book is for you.

Just go to http://bit.ly/superfoods-gift

www.ingramcontent.com/pod-product-compliance
Lightning Source LLC
Chambersburg PA
CBHW060933220326
41597CB00020BA/3727